The Wheat

Revolution

The Shocking Truth About Our #1 Food Addiction

Dr. Myles Watson Collins

Dear Readers,

If you enjoyed reading and using this book, please leave a review. Your feedback means a lot to me and helps others discover the book. I will really appreciate it.

Thank you!

Contents

Introduction

The Turning Point: Dr. Myles Watson Collins's Personal Journey

Imagine waking up every morning with a foggy mind, persistent fatigue, and a stomach that never seems to settle. This was my life for years. Despite being a nutritionist with a deep understanding of dietary principles, I was constantly battling unexplained health issues. I meticulously followed a balanced diet, exercised regularly, and took all the recommended supplements, yet something was not right. My energy levels were plummeting, my concentration was shot, and I felt an underlying sense of discomfort every single day.

One afternoon, while reading through the latest research on diet-related health issues, I stumbled upon a study linking wheat consumption to various health problems, including those I was experiencing. Intrigued, I delved deeper into the subject. The more I read, the more I recognized my symptoms in the stories of others who had struggled with wheat. Despite my initial skepticism—I had always believed wheat to be a healthy, essential part of the diet—I decided to experiment on myself. I eliminated wheat from my meals entirely.

The first few days were rough. I experienced headaches, cravings, and mood swings. But by the end of the first week, something miraculous began to happen. The fog in my mind started to lift. I woke up with more energy. My digestive issues began to resolve. I felt a clarity and vitality that I hadn't experienced in years. This was my turning point.

Realizing the profound impact that removing wheat had on my health, I knew I had to share this discovery. Thus began my journey into researching the hidden dangers of modern wheat and how it affects our bodies and minds. The result of that research is this book, "The Wheat Revolution: The Shocking Truth About Our #1 Food Addiction."

The Hidden Truth Behind Wheat

For thousands of years, wheat has been a staple in human diets. It's deeply ingrained in our culinary traditions and cultural practices. From bread and pasta to cakes and cookies, wheat is ubiquitous. Yet, what if I told you that the wheat we consume today is vastly different from the ancient grains our ancestors ate? Modern wheat has undergone significant changes through selective breeding and industrial processing, making it a far cry from its original form.

These changes have serious implications for our health. Modern wheat is not only nutritionally inferior but also has properties that can trigger inflammation, weight gain, and a host of chronic diseases. The rise of gluten-related disorders, the obesity epidemic, and increasing mental health issues can all be linked to our consumption of wheat.

In "The Wheat Revolution," we delve into the science behind these claims, providing you with a clear understanding of how wheat affects your body and mind. We explore the journey of wheat from ancient grains to the high-yield, nutrient-depleted versions we see today. We examine the addictive nature of wheat and how it can lead to overeating and cravings. We also look at the connection between wheat and various chronic diseases, including diabetes, heart disease, and autoimmune disorders.

Why This Book Matters

This book is not just another diet book. It's a comprehensive guide to understanding the profound impact wheat has on your health and well-being. It's about empowering you with knowledge and tools to make informed dietary choices that can transform your life. By the end of this book, you will understand why wheat might be the culprit behind many of your health issues and how you can reclaim your health by making simple yet powerful changes to your diet.

Whether you're struggling with unexplained health problems, looking to lose weight, or simply want to feel better, this book is for you. The information and strategies provided here are backed by scientific research and real-life case studies, including my own personal journey. You'll learn how to identify hidden sources of wheat, find suitable substitutes, and navigate the challenges of a wheat-free lifestyle. You'll also discover the long-term health benefits of eliminating wheat and how to maintain a balanced, nutritious diet without it.

As you read through this book, I encourage you to keep an open mind and be willing to experiment with your diet. The goal is not just to eliminate wheat but to understand how your body responds to different foods and to find a diet that truly supports your health and well-being.

Consider this book your roadmap to a healthier, happier life. Take the first step by diving into the pages that follow. Learn about the hidden dangers of wheat, explore the science behind it, and discover how you can break free from the grip of wheat addiction. Your journey to better health starts here.

Embark on this journey with me and discover the transformative power of a wheat-free life. Together, we can uncover the hidden truth about wheat and pave the way for a healthier, happier future. Let's take this step towards optimal health and well-being—starting today.

Chapter 1

The History of Wheat: From Ancient Grain to Modern Menace

Introduction to Wheat's Journey

Wheat, one of the most ancient and significant crops in human history, has played a crucial role in the development of civilizations. Its journey from wild grass to a staple food source spans thousands of years and reflects the ingenuity and adaptability of human societies. This chapter explores the origins of wheat, its evolution through the ages, and how it has become a central component of the modern diet. We will examine the transformation of wheat cultivation practices, the impact of the Green Revolution, and the shift from whole grains to refined products. By understanding the history of wheat, we can better appreciate its current status and the implications for our health.

Brief Overview of Wheat's Origins in Ancient Civilizations

Wheat's story begins in the Fertile Crescent, a region in the Middle East often considered the cradle of civilization. Around 10,000 years ago, early agricultural societies began domesticating wild grasses, leading to the cultivation of wheat. This marked a significant shift from nomadic lifestyles to settled farming communities.

The Early Days of Domestication

Wild Grasses to Cultivated Wheat: The ancestors of modern wheat, such as einkorn and emmer, were wild grasses. Early farmers selectively bred these plants for desirable traits, such as larger seeds and easier threshing, leading to the first domesticated wheat varieties.

Agricultural Revolution: The domestication of wheat contributed to the

Neolithic Agricultural Revolution. It allowed humans to produce surplus food, supporting larger populations and the development of complex societies.

Wheat in Ancient Civilizations

Mesopotamia: In Mesopotamia, wheat became a staple crop, integral to the diet and economy. The Sumerians, Akkadians, and Babylonians cultivated wheat extensively, using it to make bread and beer, which were central to their culture and religion.

Ancient Egypt: Wheat was also fundamental in ancient Egypt. The Egyptians mastered irrigation techniques, allowing them to grow wheat in the fertile Nile Delta. Wheat was used to make bread, a primary food source, and was even used as currency and an offering to the gods.

Greece and Rome: In classical antiquity, wheat continued to be a dietary staple. The Greeks and Romans not only consumed wheat but also traded it, spreading its cultivation throughout Europe.

Cultural Significance

Religious and Symbolic Role: Wheat held a symbolic and religious significance in many ancient cultures. It was often associated with fertility and prosperity. In ancient Greek mythology, Demeter, the goddess of the harvest, was often depicted with sheaves of wheat.

Economic Impact: The ability to cultivate and store wheat led to the development of trade and commerce. Surpluses could be traded for other goods, contributing to the rise of complex economies.

Evolution of Wheat Cultivation and Consumption

As human societies evolved, so did their agricultural practices. The cultivation and consumption of wheat underwent significant changes, influenced by technological advancements, environmental factors, and cultural shifts.

Advancements in Agricultural Techniques

Selective Breeding: Early farmers practiced selective breeding, choosing plants with desirable traits such as higher yields and better resistance to pests and diseases. This led to the development of various wheat varieties adapted to different climates and soils.

Irrigation and Plowing: The invention of irrigation systems and the plow revolutionized agriculture. These innovations allowed farmers to cultivate larger areas of land and increase productivity.

Wheat Spreads Across Continents

Expansion of Cultivation: As civilizations expanded, so did wheat cultivation. Trade routes, such as the Silk Road, facilitated the spread of wheat to Asia, Africa, and Europe. Each region adapted wheat cultivation to its specific environmental conditions.

Adaptation to Local Climates: Different regions developed unique wheat varieties suited to their climates. For example, durum wheat, used to make pasta, thrives in the Mediterranean climate, while hard red winter wheat is well-suited to the Great Plains of North America.

Culinary Evolution

Ancient Recipes: The ways in which wheat was consumed also evolved. Ancient recipes from Mesopotamia, Egypt, Greece, and Rome reveal a rich culinary history involving various forms of bread, porridge, and beer.

Bread as a Staple: Over time, bread became the primary way to consume wheat. Techniques for leavening bread improved, leading to a variety of bread types, from flatbreads to fluffy loaves.

Transformation through the Ages

The cultivation and consumption of wheat continued to evolve, particularly during the Middle Ages and the Renaissance, as agricultural practices improved and trade expanded. However, the most dramatic changes occurred in the 20th century.

Medieval and Renaissance Agriculture

Feudal Systems and Crop Rotation: During the Middle Ages, the feudal system dictated agricultural practices. Crop rotation and the three-field system became common, improving soil fertility and wheat yields.

Trade and Exploration: The Renaissance period saw an increase in trade and exploration, leading to the exchange of agricultural knowledge and techniques. European explorers introduced wheat to the Americas, where it became a key crop.

The Green Revolution

Technological Advancements: The 20th century brought significant technological advancements in agriculture, known as the Green Revolution. This period saw the development of high-yield wheat varieties, advanced irrigation techniques, and the use of chemical fertilizers and pesticides.

High-Yield Dwarf Wheat: One of the most significant developments was the creation of high-yield dwarf wheat by agronomist Norman Borlaug in the 1960s. This variety was shorter and sturdier, allowing it to support larger grain heads and resist lodging (falling over). It significantly increased wheat production, particularly in developing countries.

Global Impact: The Green Revolution transformed global agriculture, alleviating food shortages and reducing hunger in many parts of the world. However, it also led to the widespread use of chemical inputs and monoculture farming, raising concerns about environmental sustainability and biodiversity.

Wheat in the Modern Diet

The modern era has seen a profound transformation in how wheat is consumed. From whole grains to highly processed products, wheat has become ubiquitous in the contemporary diet.

Introduction of Wheat in Processed Foods

Industrialization of Food Production: The industrialization of food production in the 20th century led to the creation of a vast array of processed foods. Wheat became a key ingredient in many of these products due to its versatility and availability.

Convenience Foods: The rise of convenience foods, such as ready-to-eat meals, snacks, and fast food, often relies heavily on wheat. Wheat flour is used in everything from bread and pasta to pastries, cereals, and snacks.

Additives and Preservatives: Processed wheat products often contain additives and preservatives to enhance flavor, texture, and shelf life. This has led to the widespread consumption of refined wheat products that are far removed from their whole grain origins.

Shift from Whole Grains to Refined Products

Refining Process: The refining process strips wheat of its bran and germ, leaving primarily the starchy endosperm. This process removes many of the nutrients, including fiber, vitamins, and minerals, resulting in a product that is less nutritious than whole grain wheat.

Health Implications: The shift from whole grains to refined wheat products has been linked to various health issues, including obesity, diabetes, and cardiovascular diseases. Refined wheat has a higher glycemic index, leading to rapid spikes in blood sugar levels.

Cultural and Economic Factors

Cultural Preferences: Cultural preferences and marketing have played significant roles in the shift towards refined wheat products. White bread, for example, was once considered a status symbol, leading to its widespread popularity.

Economic Considerations: Refined wheat products are often cheaper to produce and have a longer shelf life than whole grain products. This makes them more economically attractive for both producers and consumers.

Summary of Historical Impact

The history of wheat, from its ancient origins to its modern status, reflects a complex journey marked by innovation, adaptation, and transformation. The evolution of wheat cultivation practices and consumption patterns has had profound implications for human health and society.

Nutritional Profile and Health Effects

Ancient vs. Modern Wheat: Ancient wheat varieties, such as einkorn and emmer, were nutritionally dense and consumed in their whole grain form. Modern wheat, particularly refined products, lacks many of the essential nutrients found in its ancient counterparts.

Health Consequences: The widespread consumption of refined wheat products has been associated with various health issues, including obesity, diabetes, and cardiovascular diseases. The rise of gluten-related disorders, such as celiac disease and non-celiac gluten sensitivity, further highlights the health implications of modern wheat.

Cultural and Economic Influence

Role in Civilization: Wheat has played a pivotal role in the development of human civilizations, supporting population growth and the rise of complex societies. It has been a cornerstone of economies, cultures, and religious practices.

Modern Challenges: Today, the dominance of wheat in the global diet presents challenges related to health, sustainability, and food security. The environmental impact of large-scale wheat cultivation, the loss of biodiversity, and the rise of monoculture farming are pressing concerns.

Looking Ahead

Future of Wheat: The future of wheat will depend on addressing these challenges. Sustainable farming practices, the promotion of whole grain consumption, and the development of wheat varieties that balance productivity with nutritional quality are essential steps.

Personal Choices: On an individual level, understanding the history and impact of wheat can inform dietary choices. Opting for whole grain products and reducing reliance on highly processed foods can contribute to better health outcomes.

In all, the journey of wheat from an ancient grain to a modern menace underscores the importance of re-evaluating our relationship with this staple crop. By learning from its history, we can make informed choices that promote both personal health and the sustainability of our food systems.

Chapter 2

Understanding Wheat Addiction

What is Food Addiction?

Food addiction is a concept that describes an uncontrollable desire to consume certain foods despite negative consequences. This phenomenon can be compared to other forms of addiction, such as those to drugs or alcohol, where the individual continues the behavior despite knowing it can cause harm. In this chapter, we will delve into the nature of food addiction, focusing particularly on how wheat can become an addictive substance.

Explanation of Food Addiction and Its Criteria

Food addiction can be characterized by several key criteria:

1. **Cravings**: An intense desire to eat specific foods, even when not physically hungry.
2. **Loss of Control**: Inability to stop eating or limit the amount consumed, even when trying to cut down.
3. **Continued Use Despite Negative Consequences**: Persisting in eating behaviors that lead to health problems, weight gain, or emotional distress.
4. **Tolerance**: Needing to eat more of the food to experience the same satisfaction.
5. **Withdrawal**: Experiencing negative physical or emotional symptoms when not eating the addictive food.

These criteria are similar to those used to diagnose substance use disorders, highlighting the parallels between food addiction and other types of addiction.

Comparison to Other Forms of Addiction

Food addiction shares many similarities with addictions to substances like drugs and alcohol:

- **Brain Chemistry**: Both types of addiction involve changes in the brain's reward system. Foods, particularly those high in sugar, fat, or refined carbohydrates like wheat, can stimulate the release of dopamine, a neurotransmitter associated with pleasure and reward.
- **Behavioral Patterns**: Addictive behaviors in both food and substance addictions include binging, loss of control, and prioritizing the addictive substance over other activities or responsibilities.
- **Withdrawal and Tolerance**: Just as with drugs or alcohol, individuals addicted to certain foods may experience withdrawal symptoms when they stop consuming them and may require larger amounts to achieve the same effects over time.

The Science of Wheat Addiction

The addictive potential of wheat can be traced to its biochemical properties. Wheat contains compounds that can affect the brain and body in ways that promote addiction.

Biochemical Pathways Involved in Wheat Consumption and Addiction

When we eat wheat, our bodies break it down into its component nutrients. However, wheat also contains specific proteins and compounds that can influence brain chemistry:

1. **Gluten**: The primary protein in wheat, gluten, is broken down into smaller peptides called exorphins during digestion.
2. **Exorphins**: These peptides can cross the blood-brain barrier and bind to opioid receptors in the brain, producing effects similar to those of opiate drugs, such as a sense of pleasure and reduced pain.

The Role of Gliadin and Exorphins in Stimulating Appetite and Cravings

1. **Gliadin**: A component of gluten, gliadin can stimulate appetite. Research has shown that gliadin peptides can bind to opioid receptors in the brain, leading to increased hunger and cravings. This effect is particularly potent because it directly influences the brain's reward and pleasure centers.
2. **Exorphins**: The exorphins produced from gluten digestion can produce addictive-like effects by binding to the brain's opioid receptors. This binding creates feelings of euphoria and pleasure, similar to those produced by narcotic drugs. This can lead to a cycle of craving and consumption that mirrors other forms of addiction.

Personal Stories of Addiction

Hearing from individuals who have struggled with wheat addiction can provide valuable insight into the reality of this condition. These personal stories highlight the challenges and triumphs of those who have battled with their dependency on wheat.

Case Studies and Anecdotes from Individuals Battling Wheat Addiction

Case Study 1: Brenda's Battle with Bread

Brenda, a 35-year-old mother of two, struggled with her weight for years. Despite trying numerous diets, she found it nearly impossible to cut back on bread and pasta. She often felt uncontrollable cravings for these foods, leading to binge-eating episodes that left her feeling guilty and depressed. After learning about wheat addiction, Brenda decided to eliminate wheat from her diet. The first few weeks were tough, with intense cravings and mood swings, but she eventually noticed significant improvements in her energy levels and mood. Brenda's story illustrates the powerful grip wheat can have and the positive changes that can occur when breaking free from its hold.

Case Study 2: Mark's Struggle with Wheat Withdrawal

Mark, a 42-year-old office worker, experienced severe digestive issues and chronic fatigue. After multiple doctor visits and tests, he was advised to try a gluten-free diet. Initially skeptical, Mark decided to give it a try. The withdrawal symptoms were challenging—headaches, irritability, and intense cravings—but after a month, Mark noticed remarkable improvements in his symptoms. His digestive issues resolved, and he felt more energetic and focused. Mark's journey underscores the physical and psychological withdrawal symptoms associated with wheat addiction and the potential health benefits of eliminating wheat.

Case Study 3: Kathleen's Emotional Rollercoaster

Kathleen, a college student, found solace in comfort foods like cookies, cakes, and pasta during stressful periods. She noticed that her cravings for these foods intensified during exams or emotional distress. After learning about the addictive properties of wheat, Kathleen realized that her reliance on these foods was more than just a coping mechanism—it was an addiction. With the support of a nutritionist and counselor, Kathleen gradually reduced her wheat intake. She experienced mood swings and cravings initially but eventually found healthier ways to manage stress. Kathleen's experience highlights the emotional component of wheat addiction and the importance of support in overcoming it.

Recognizing the Signs

Identifying wheat addiction can be challenging, as it often manifests in subtle ways. However, recognizing the signs can help individuals understand their relationship with wheat and take steps towards addressing it.

Symptoms and Behaviors Indicative of Wheat Addiction

1. **Constant Cravings**: Persistent and intense cravings for wheat-based products, even when not physically hungry.
2. **Overeating**: Consuming large quantities of wheat-based foods in one sitting, often feeling unable to stop despite feeling full.
3. **Emotional Eating**: Turning to wheat-based comfort foods during times of stress, anxiety, or emotional distress.
4. **Guilt and Regret**: Feeling guilty or regretful after eating wheat-based

foods, but continuing to eat them despite these feelings.

5. **Physical Symptoms**: Experiencing physical symptoms such as bloating, headaches, or fatigue after consuming wheat, yet continuing to eat it.

6. **Failed Attempts to Cut Down**: Trying to reduce or eliminate wheat from the diet but repeatedly failing due to strong cravings or withdrawal symptoms.

7. **Preoccupation with Wheat**: Spending a significant amount of time thinking about, obtaining, or consuming wheat-based foods.

Understanding these signs and acknowledging the potential for addiction is the first step towards addressing the issue. In the following chapters, we will explore strategies and solutions for overcoming wheat addiction, promoting better health and well-being.

Wheat addiction is a complex and multifaceted condition, deeply rooted in both our biology and culture. By understanding the science behind wheat's addictive properties, recognizing the signs of addiction, and learning from personal stories, we can begin to address this issue more effectively. The journey to overcoming wheat addiction is challenging, but with the right knowledge and support, it is possible to break free and achieve better health.

Chapter 3

The Hidden Dangers of Modern Wheat

Wheat has been a cornerstone of the human diet for thousands of years, providing essential nutrients and calories to sustain populations. However, modern wheat, significantly altered from its ancient ancestors, poses hidden dangers that affect our health. This chapter explores the nutritional degradation of modern wheat, its links to chronic diseases, and the ongoing gluten controversy.

Nutritional Degradation

Modern wheat has undergone extensive changes due to selective breeding, agricultural practices, and industrial processing. These changes have significantly affected its nutritional profile.

The Loss of Nutrients in Modern Wheat Compared to Ancient Varieties

Ancient wheat varieties such as einkorn, emmer, and spelt were nutritionally rich. They contained higher levels of protein, fiber, vitamins, and minerals compared to modern wheat. Over time, the focus on high-yield, disease-resistant strains has led to the reduction of these essential nutrients.

1. **Protein Content**: Ancient wheat varieties had a higher protein content, contributing to better muscle maintenance and overall health. Modern wheat has lower protein levels, affecting the quality of protein intake.
2. **Fiber**: Fiber is crucial for digestive health and preventing chronic diseases. Ancient wheat was rich in fiber, while modern wheat has significantly less due to selective breeding and processing.
3. **Vitamins and Minerals**: Ancient wheat was a good source of vitamins

and minerals such as B vitamins, iron, magnesium, and zinc. Modern wheat has lower levels of these nutrients, contributing to potential deficiencies in populations that rely heavily on wheat-based products.

Impact of Refining and Processing on Wheat's Nutritional Content

The refining process further depletes the nutritional value of wheat. Refined wheat flour, commonly used in many processed foods, is stripped of its bran and germ, leaving primarily the starchy endosperm. This process removes most of the fiber, vitamins, and minerals, resulting in a product that is calorie-dense but nutrient-poor.

1. **Loss of Fiber**: The removal of bran during refining significantly reduces the fiber content of wheat, impacting digestive health and increasing the risk of conditions such as

constipation, diverticulosis, and colorectal cancer.

2. **Depletion of Nutrients**: The refining process removes essential nutrients, leading to a reliance on fortified foods to meet dietary needs. However, these fortifications do not fully replicate the natural nutrient profile of whole grains.

3. **Increased Glycemic Index**: Refined wheat products have a higher glycemic index, causing rapid spikes in blood sugar levels. This can lead to insulin resistance, increased hunger, and a higher risk of developing type 2 diabetes.

Wheat and Chronic Diseases

The consumption of modern wheat is linked to several chronic diseases, including obesity, diabetes, heart disease, and various inflammatory and autoimmune disorders.

Links Between Wheat Consumption and Conditions Like Obesity, Diabetes, and Heart Disease

Modern wheat's high glycemic index and refined nature contribute to weight gain and metabolic disorders.

1. **Obesity**: Refined wheat products are calorie-dense and low in fiber, leading to overconsumption and weight gain. The high glycemic index of these foods causes rapid spikes and crashes in blood sugar, resulting in increased hunger and overeating.
2. **Diabetes**: The consumption of high-glycemic foods, such as refined wheat, contributes to insulin resistance and the development of type 2 diabetes. Frequent blood sugar spikes stress the pancreas, leading to impaired insulin function over time.
3. **Heart Disease**: Diets high in refined wheat are linked to higher levels of triglycerides and low-density lipoprotein (LDL) cholesterol,

increasing the risk of heart disease. The lack of fiber also contributes to poor cardiovascular health.

Inflammatory Responses and Autoimmune Disorders Associated with Wheat

Modern wheat can trigger inflammatory responses and contribute to autoimmune disorders in susceptible individuals.

1. **Inflammation**: The gliadin protein in wheat can cause inflammation in the gut, leading to increased intestinal permeability, commonly known as "leaky gut." This allows toxins and undigested food particles to enter the bloodstream, triggering systemic inflammation.
2. **Autoimmune Disorders**: Wheat consumption is linked to autoimmune conditions such as celiac disease, rheumatoid arthritis, and Hashimoto's thyroiditis. In genetically predisposed individuals, wheat proteins can trigger

an immune response that attacks the body's tissues.

The Gluten Controversy

Gluten, a protein found in wheat, barley, and rye, has become a controversial topic due to its association with various health conditions. Understanding the differences between celiac disease, gluten sensitivity, and wheat allergy is crucial for addressing the gluten controversy.

Differences Between Celiac Disease, Gluten Sensitivity, and Wheat Allergy

1. **Celiac Disease**: Celiac disease is an autoimmune disorder in which the ingestion of gluten triggers an immune response that damages the lining of the small intestine. This damage impairs nutrient absorption and can lead to various symptoms such as diarrhea, weight loss, and fatigue. A strict gluten-free diet is necessary to manage the condition.

2. **Gluten Sensitivity**: Non-celiac gluten sensitivity (NCGS) refers to a condition where individuals experience symptoms similar to celiac disease upon consuming gluten but do not have the same intestinal damage or autoimmune markers. Symptoms can include bloating, abdominal pain, headache, and fatigue. While the exact cause is not well understood, a gluten-free diet often alleviates symptoms.

3. **Wheat Allergy**: Wheat allergy is an allergic reaction to proteins found in wheat, not just gluten. Symptoms can range from mild (hives, itching) to severe (anaphylaxis). Avoiding wheat and wheat-containing products is essential for managing the allergy.

The Rise of Gluten-Free Diets and Their Implications

The popularity of gluten-free diets has surged in recent years, driven by increased awareness of gluten-related disorders and the perceived health benefits of avoiding gluten.

1. **Health Trends**: Many people adopt gluten-free diets without a medical diagnosis, believing it to be healthier or beneficial for weight loss. While a gluten-free diet is essential for those with celiac disease or gluten sensitivity, it is not inherently healthier for the general population.

2. **Nutritional Considerations**: Gluten-free diets can be nutritionally adequate if well-planned, but they may lack essential nutrients found in whole grains, such as fiber, iron, and B vitamins. It's important for those on gluten-free diets to find alternative sources of these nutrients.

3. **Market Growth**: The demand for gluten-free products has led to a growing market of gluten-free foods. However, many of these products are highly processed and may contain unhealthy additives or higher levels of sugar and fat to compensate for the texture and taste of gluten.

The hidden dangers of modern wheat stem from its nutritional degradation, links to chronic diseases, and the ongoing gluten controversy. Understanding these issues can help individuals make informed dietary choices and consider alternatives that promote better health. As we continue to learn more about wheat's impact on our bodies, it becomes increasingly clear that the way we consume and process wheat needs to be re-evaluated for the sake of our health and well-being.

Chapter 4

Wheat's Role in the Obesity Epidemic

Wheat, a staple in many diets worldwide, has been linked to the rising obesity epidemic. This chapter explores how wheat contributes to weight gain, the mechanisms behind its effects on the body, and strategies for breaking the cycle of wheat-induced obesity.

Caloric Density and Weight Gain

Wheat plays a significant role in our diets, but its contribution to caloric intake and weight gain cannot be overlooked.

How Wheat Contributes to Increased Calorie Intake

Wheat is present in many foods, especially processed ones. These products are often high in calories but low in essential nutrients.

1. **Wheat in Processed Foods**: Many processed foods, like bread, pasta, cereals, and snacks, are made from wheat. These foods are often calorie-dense, meaning they provide a lot of calories in a small portion. Consuming these foods regularly can lead to a high calorie intake.

2. **Portion Sizes**: Wheat-based foods are often eaten in large portions. For example, it's easy to consume several slices of bread or a large bowl of pasta in one sitting. This leads to consuming more calories than necessary.

3. **Hidden Calories**: Wheat is also found in many foods where you might not expect it, such as sauces, soups, and processed meats. These hidden sources of wheat add to overall calorie intake.

The Glycemic Index of Wheat Products and Its Effect on Blood Sugar Levels

The glycemic index (GI) measures how quickly a food raises blood sugar levels. Wheat products often have a high GI, which affects blood sugar and insulin levels.

1. **High Glycemic Index**: Foods made from refined wheat, like white bread and pasta, have a high GI. This means they are quickly broken down into glucose, leading to rapid spikes in blood sugar levels.
2. **Blood Sugar Spikes and Crashes**: When blood sugar levels spike, the body releases insulin to bring them back down. This can lead to a rapid drop in blood sugar, causing feelings of hunger and leading to overeating.
3. **Insulin Response**: High GI foods cause a strong insulin response. Insulin is a hormone that helps store glucose as fat. Frequent spikes in insulin can lead to increased fat

storage, especially in the abdominal area.

Insulin Resistance and Fat Storage

Wheat consumption can contribute to insulin resistance and increased fat storage, both of which are linked to obesity.

The Connection Between Wheat Consumption and Insulin Resistance

Insulin resistance occurs when cells in the body become less responsive to insulin, leading to higher blood sugar levels and increased fat storage.

1. **Chronic High Insulin Levels**: Regular consumption of high-GI wheat products can keep insulin levels elevated. Over time, this can lead to insulin resistance, where cells no longer respond effectively to insulin.
2. **Fat Storage**: When insulin resistance develops, the body stores more fat, particularly around the abdomen. This type of fat storage is associated with

an increased risk of obesity-related diseases, such as type 2 diabetes and cardiovascular disease.

Mechanisms Behind Wheat-Induced Weight Gain

Several mechanisms explain how wheat contributes to weight gain.

1. **Appetite Stimulation**: Wheat contains compounds like gliadin, which can stimulate appetite and lead to increased food intake. This makes it harder to control portions and caloric intake.
2. **Addictive Properties**: Wheat can have addictive properties, leading to cravings and overconsumption. The exorphins produced from gluten digestion can bind to opioid receptors in the brain, creating a sense of pleasure and reward similar to addictive substances.
3. **Increased Fat Storage**: As mentioned earlier, high insulin levels

promote fat storage. Additionally, the rapid digestion of refined wheat leads to quick energy availability, which, if not used, is stored as fat.

Breaking the Cycle

Reducing wheat consumption can help break the cycle of weight gain and promote better health.

Strategies to Reduce Wheat Consumption and Promote Weight Loss

Here are some practical strategies to help reduce wheat intake and encourage weight loss:

1. **Choose Whole Grains**: Opt for whole grain alternatives to refined wheat products. Whole grains contain more fiber and nutrients, which can help control blood sugar levels and reduce hunger.

Examples include whole wheat bread, brown rice, quinoa, and oats.

2. **Read Labels**: Be aware of hidden sources of wheat in processed foods. Check ingredient labels and choose products that are free from refined wheat.
3. **Increase Fiber Intake**: Foods high in fiber can help you feel full longer and reduce overall calorie intake.

Example include vegetables, fruits, legumes, and whole grains in your diet.

4. **Healthy Substitutes**: Use alternatives to wheat-based products. For example, use lettuce wraps instead of bread, or try spiralized vegetables instead of pasta.
5. **Mindful Eating**: Pay attention to portion sizes and avoid overeating. Eating slowly and savoring your food can help you recognize when you're full.

6. **Balanced Diet**: Ensure your diet is balanced with a variety of nutrients. Include lean proteins, healthy fats, and plenty of fruits and vegetables.
7. **Avoid Processed Foods**: Limit consumption of processed foods, which are often high in refined wheat and added sugars. Choose whole, minimally processed foods instead.
8. **Stay Hydrated**: Drinking water can help control hunger and reduce the likelihood of overeating.

By implementing these strategies, you can reduce your dependence on wheat, decrease caloric intake, and promote healthier eating habits. This approach not only supports weight loss but also improves overall health and well-being.

Wheat plays a significant role in the obesity epidemic due to its high caloric density, effects on blood sugar levels, and contribution to insulin resistance and fat storage. By understanding these mechanisms and implementing strategies to reduce wheat consumption, individuals can break the cycle of weight gain and improve their health. Making mindful food choices and prioritizing whole, nutrient-dense foods can lead to lasting positive changes in weight and overall well-being.

Chapter 5

Wheat and Mental Health

Impact on the Brain

Wheat has been a staple in human diets for thousands of years, but its effects on mental health are becoming a growing concern. This chapter explores how wheat consumption can affect cognitive function, mental clarity, and the potential links between wheat and neurological disorders.

How Wheat Consumption Affects Cognitive Function and Mental Clarity

Wheat can influence brain health in several ways, impacting cognitive function and mental clarity.

1. **Gluten and Brain Function**: Gluten, a protein found in wheat, can affect the brain. For some individuals, gluten can lead to inflammation and impair brain function, causing brain

fog, difficulty concentrating, and reduced mental clarity.

2. **Blood Sugar Spikes and Crashes**: Wheat products, especially those made from refined flour, have a high glycemic index. This causes rapid spikes in blood sugar levels followed by crashes. These fluctuations can lead to feelings of fatigue, irritability, and difficulty focusing.

3. **Inflammation**: Chronic inflammation in the body can affect the brain. Some studies suggest that gluten can contribute to inflammation, which may impair cognitive function and lead to symptoms such as brain fog and forgetfulness.

Links Between Wheat and Neurological Disorders

Research has begun to uncover potential links between wheat consumption and various neurological disorders.

1. **Celiac Disease and Neurological Symptoms**: Celiac disease is an autoimmune condition triggered by gluten. In addition to digestive symptoms, celiac disease can cause neurological symptoms such as headaches, peripheral neuropathy (nerve damage), and ataxia (loss of coordination).
2. **Gluten Ataxia**: Gluten ataxia is a specific neurological condition where gluten consumption leads to damage in the cerebellum, the part of the brain that controls coordination. This can result in difficulty walking, poor balance, and coordination problems.
3. **Non-Celiac Gluten Sensitivity**: Some individuals experience neurological symptoms when

consuming gluten, even if they do not have celiac disease. Symptoms can include headaches, brain fog, and mood disturbances.

4. **Autoimmune Disorders**: Wheat consumption has been linked to various autoimmune disorders, which can have neurological implications. For example, multiple sclerosis (MS) and other autoimmune conditions can cause neurological symptoms that may be exacerbated by gluten.

Mood Disorders and Wheat

Wheat consumption has been linked to mood disorders such as depression, anxiety, and mood swings. This section explores these connections and provides case studies and scientific research on wheat's psychological impact.

The Connection Between Wheat Consumption and Depression, Anxiety, and Mood Swings

1. **Depression**: Some studies suggest that gluten can contribute to depression. For individuals with gluten sensitivity or celiac disease, consuming gluten can trigger an immune response that affects the brain and mood.
2. **Anxiety**: Gluten has been linked to anxiety in some individuals. The inflammation and immune response triggered by gluten can affect neurotransmitter function, leading to increased anxiety.
3. **Mood Swings**: The blood sugar fluctuations caused by high-glycemic wheat products can lead to mood swings. Rapid changes in blood sugar levels can cause irritability, anger, and emotional instability.

Case Studies and Scientific Research on Wheat's Psychological Impact

Case Study 1: Carolina's Struggle with Depression

Carolina, a 28-year-old teacher, experienced chronic depression and anxiety. After numerous treatments and medications, she decided to try a gluten-free diet. Within weeks, she noticed a significant improvement in her mood and energy levels. Her depression symptoms decreased, and she felt more emotionally stable. Carolina's case highlights the potential link between gluten and mood disorders.

Case Study 2: John's Battle with Anxiety

John, a 35-year-old software engineer, suffered from severe anxiety and panic attacks. He eliminated gluten from his diet after reading about its potential effects on mental health. Over time, John's anxiety levels decreased, and he experienced fewer panic attacks. John's experience suggests that gluten might play a role in exacerbating anxiety for some individuals.

Scientific Research

- **Study on Celiac Disease and Depression**: A study published in the journal "Gastroenterology" found that individuals with celiac disease are at a higher risk of developing depression and anxiety. The researchers suggested that the immune response and inflammation caused by gluten could contribute to these mood disorders.
- **Gluten Sensitivity and Mental Health**: Research published in "Psychiatry Research" indicated that individuals with non-celiac gluten sensitivity reported significant improvements in mood and mental health after adopting a gluten-free diet. This study supports the idea that gluten can affect mental health in people without celiac disease.

Improving Mental Health through Diet

Dietary changes can play a crucial role in improving mental health and alleviating wheat-induced issues. This section outlines dietary strategies to enhance mental well-being.

Dietary Changes That Can Alleviate Wheat-Induced Mental Health Issues

1. **Eliminate Gluten**: For individuals who suspect gluten might be affecting their mental health, eliminating gluten from the diet is the first step. This involves avoiding wheat, barley, rye, and any products containing these grains.
2. **Choose Whole Foods**: Focus on whole, minimally processed foods that provide essential nutrients for brain health. These include fruits, vegetables, lean proteins, nuts, seeds, and healthy fats.
3. **Increase Omega-3 Fatty Acids**: Omega-3 fatty acids, found in fish,

flaxseeds, and walnuts, are crucial for brain health. They can help reduce inflammation and support cognitive function and mood.

4. **Boost Antioxidants**: Foods rich in antioxidants, such as berries, dark leafy greens, and nuts, can help protect the brain from oxidative stress and inflammation.

5. **Maintain Stable Blood Sugar Levels**: Avoid high-glycemic foods that cause rapid blood sugar spikes. Choose low-glycemic options such as whole grains, legumes, and non-starchy vegetables to maintain stable blood sugar levels and prevent mood swings.

6. **Consider Probiotics**: The gut-brain connection is well-established, and maintaining a healthy gut can support mental health. Probiotic-rich foods like yogurt, kefir, sauerkraut, and kimchi can promote a healthy gut microbiome.

7. **Stay Hydrated**: Dehydration can affect mood and cognitive function. Ensure adequate water intake throughout the day to support overall mental health.

8. **Monitor Nutrient Intake**: Ensure adequate intake of key nutrients for brain health, including B vitamins, magnesium, zinc, and iron. These nutrients play a role in neurotransmitter function and mental well-being.

The consumption of wheat can have significant effects on mental health, impacting cognitive function, mood, and neurological health. By understanding these effects and making informed dietary choices, individuals can improve their mental well-being and alleviate wheat-induced mental health issues. Prioritizing a balanced diet rich in whole foods, essential nutrients, and healthy fats can support optimal brain function and emotional stability.

Chapter 6

The Inflammation Connection

Inflammatory Mechanisms of Wheat

Wheat is a staple food for many people worldwide, but it can also be a significant contributor to inflammation in the body. Understanding how wheat triggers inflammatory processes is crucial for addressing health issues related to chronic inflammation.

How Wheat Triggers Inflammatory Processes in the Body

Wheat contains several components that can stimulate inflammation. Two of the most significant are gluten and lectins.

1. **Gluten**: Gluten is a protein found in wheat, barley, and rye. For some people, gluten can be highly inflammatory. When these individuals

consume gluten, their immune systems mistakenly identify it as a harmful substance, leading to an immune response that causes inflammation. This is particularly evident in people with celiac disease, where gluten triggers an autoimmune response that damages the lining of the small intestine.

2. **Lectins**: Lectins are proteins found in many plants, including wheat. They can bind to carbohydrates on cell surfaces, which can disrupt cellular communication and lead to inflammation. Lectins are resistant to digestion, meaning they can remain intact as they pass through the digestive system, potentially causing harm.

3. **Amylase-Trypsin Inhibitors (ATIs)**: ATIs are proteins in wheat that can trigger an inflammatory response in the gut. They can interfere with digestive enzymes, leading to

inflammation and digestive discomfort.

The Role of Lectins and Gluten in Inflammation

1. **Lectins**: Lectins in wheat can bind to the lining of the gut, disrupting its integrity and causing a condition known as "leaky gut." This allows undigested food particles and toxins to enter the bloodstream, triggering an immune response and systemic inflammation. Chronic exposure to lectins can lead to ongoing inflammation, contributing to various health issues.
2. **Gluten**: Gluten's impact on inflammation is well-documented, especially in individuals with celiac disease or gluten sensitivity. When these individuals consume gluten, their immune systems launch an attack on the gluten proteins, leading to inflammation in the gut and other parts of the body. This chronic

inflammation can contribute to various health problems, including digestive issues, joint pain, and neurological symptoms.

Chronic Inflammation and Disease

Chronic inflammation is a prolonged, low-grade inflammatory response that can have widespread effects on the body. It is linked to many chronic diseases, and understanding this connection can help in managing these conditions.

The Link Between Chronic Inflammation and Conditions Like Arthritis, Asthma, and IBS

1. **Arthritis**: Chronic inflammation is a significant factor in arthritis, particularly rheumatoid arthritis, an autoimmune condition where the immune system attacks the joints. Wheat can exacerbate inflammation in individuals with arthritis, worsening joint pain and stiffness.

2. **Asthma**: Inflammation of the airways is a hallmark of asthma. Some studies suggest that dietary factors, including wheat consumption, can influence the severity and frequency of asthma attacks. Reducing inflammatory foods can help manage asthma symptoms.

3. **Irritable Bowel Syndrome (IBS)**: IBS is a common digestive disorder characterized by symptoms like abdominal pain, bloating, and altered bowel habits. Inflammation is believed to play a role in IBS, and for some people, wheat can trigger or worsen symptoms.

Case Studies of Individuals Experiencing Inflammation Relief After Cutting Out Wheat

Case Study 1: Michelle's Journey with Rheumatoid Arthritis

Michelle, a 45-year-old office worker, was diagnosed with rheumatoid arthritis. She experienced severe joint pain, swelling, and stiffness, which made daily tasks challenging. After researching the role of diet in inflammation, Michelle decided to eliminate wheat from her diet. Within weeks, she noticed a significant reduction in her symptoms. Her joint pain decreased, and she felt more energetic. Michelle's case highlights how removing wheat can reduce inflammation and improve quality of life for individuals with autoimmune conditions.

Case Study 2: Jason's Struggle with Asthma

Jason, a 32-year-old athlete, had struggled with asthma since childhood. His symptoms were well-managed with medication, but he still experienced frequent flare-ups that impacted his training. After consulting with a nutritionist, Jason decided to try a wheat-free diet. He noticed that his asthma symptoms improved, and he experienced fewer flare-ups. Jason's story demonstrates the potential benefits of a wheat-free diet for managing inflammatory conditions like asthma.

Case Study 3: Linda's Experience with IBS

Linda, a 28-year-old teacher, suffered from IBS. She frequently experienced bloating, abdominal pain, and irregular bowel movements. Frustrated with her symptoms, Linda decided to eliminate wheat from her diet. She found that her digestive symptoms significantly improved, and she felt more comfortable and less bloated. Linda's experience shows how dietary changes can alleviate symptoms of inflammatory digestive disorders like IBS.

Anti-Inflammatory Diets

An anti-inflammatory diet can help manage chronic inflammation and improve overall health. This section explores the foods and dietary patterns that reduce inflammation and the benefits of a wheat-free, anti-inflammatory diet.

Foods and Dietary Patterns That Reduce Inflammation

1. **Fruits and Vegetables**: Rich in antioxidants and phytochemicals, fruits and vegetables help combat inflammation. Berries, leafy greens, and cruciferous vegetables like broccoli and cauliflower are particularly effective.
2. **Healthy Fats**: Omega-3 fatty acids, found in fatty fish (like salmon and sardines), flaxseeds, and walnuts, have anti-inflammatory properties. Olive oil, rich in monounsaturated fats, also helps reduce inflammation.
3. **Whole Grains**: Instead of refined grains, choose whole grains like quinoa, brown rice, and oats, which have lower glycemic indexes and provide more fiber and nutrients.
4. **Nuts and Seeds**: Almonds, chia seeds, and sunflower seeds are excellent sources of

anti-inflammatory nutrients like vitamin E and omega-3 fatty acids.

5. **Spices and Herbs**: Turmeric, ginger, garlic, and cinnamon have anti-inflammatory properties and can enhance the flavor of meals while providing health benefits.

6. **Lean Proteins**: Opt for lean protein sources like chicken, turkey, tofu, and legumes, which support muscle health without promoting inflammation.

7. **Green Tea**: Rich in antioxidants, green tea can help reduce inflammation and provide numerous health benefits.

Benefits of a Wheat-Free, Anti-Inflammatory Diet

Adopting a wheat-free, anti-inflammatory diet can provide numerous health benefits, including reduced inflammation, improved digestion, and better overall health.

1. **Reduced Inflammation**: Eliminating wheat from the diet can help reduce

chronic inflammation, alleviating symptoms of conditions like arthritis, asthma, and IBS.

2. **Improved Digestion**: A wheat-free diet can improve digestive health by reducing bloating, gas, and abdominal pain. It can also help manage conditions like celiac disease and non-celiac gluten sensitivity.

3. **Better Mental Health**: Reducing inflammation can positively impact mental health, alleviating symptoms of depression and anxiety.

4. **Weight Management**: A diet rich in whole, anti-inflammatory foods can support healthy weight management by providing essential nutrients and promoting satiety.

5. **Enhanced Energy Levels**: Many people report increased energy and improved overall well-being after eliminating wheat and adopting an anti-inflammatory diet.

Wheat can contribute to inflammation in the body, exacerbating chronic health conditions like arthritis, asthma, and IBS. Understanding the inflammatory mechanisms of wheat and adopting an anti-inflammatory diet can help reduce inflammation and improve overall health. By choosing anti-inflammatory foods and eliminating wheat, individuals can experience significant health benefits and improved quality of life.

Chapter 7

Navigating a Wheat-Free Life

Living a wheat-free life can seem challenging, but with the right knowledge and strategies, it can lead to better health and well-being. This chapter will help you identify hidden sources of wheat, suggest substitutes and alternatives, and provide practical solutions to common challenges.

Identifying Hidden Sources of Wheat

Wheat is a common ingredient in many foods, and it can be hidden in unexpected places. Learning to identify hidden sources of wheat is crucial for maintaining a wheat-free diet.

Common Foods and Ingredients That Contain Wheat

1. **Baked Goods**: Bread, rolls, muffins, cakes, pastries, and cookies often contain wheat flour.
2. **Pasta and Noodles**: Most traditional pasta and noodles are made from wheat.
3. **Processed Foods**: Many processed foods, including soups, sauces, gravies, and dressings, may contain wheat as a thickener or filler.
4. **Snacks**: Crackers, pretzels, granola bars, and snack bars often contain wheat.
5. **Breakfast Cereals**: Many cereals, including those that are not obviously wheat-based, may contain wheat.
6. **Breading and Batter**: Fried foods, like chicken nuggets and fish sticks, often have a wheat-based coating.
7. **Condiments**: Soy sauce, teriyaki sauce, and some salad dressings may contain wheat.

8. **Beer and Malt Beverages**: Many beers are brewed with barley, which contains gluten, and some also contain wheat.

Tips for Reading Labels and Avoiding Hidden Wheat

1. **Check the Ingredients List**: Look for any mention of wheat, flour, or gluten-containing grains like barley and rye. Common ingredients that indicate the presence of wheat include:
   a. Wheat flour
   b. Durum wheat
   c. Semolina
   d. Spelt
   e. Kamut
   f. Bulgur
   g. Farina
2. **Look for Gluten-Free Labels**: Products labeled "gluten-free" are safe from wheat and other gluten-containing grains.

3. **Be Aware of Cross-Contamination**: Some products may not contain wheat but are processed in facilities that handle wheat. Check for statements about cross-contamination on labels.

4. **Familiarize Yourself with Alternative Names**: Learn the alternative names for wheat and gluten-containing ingredients. For example, "hydrolyzed vegetable protein" or "modified food starch" may contain wheat.

5. **Contact Manufacturers**: If you are unsure about a product, contact the manufacturer for more information.

Substitutes and Alternatives

Eliminating wheat from your diet doesn't mean giving up your favorite foods. Many gluten-free grains and flours can be used as substitutes in cooking and baking.

Overview of Gluten-Free Grains and Flours

Rice: A versatile and widely available grain that can be used in many dishes.

Types: White rice, brown rice, wild rice, basmati, jasmine.

Quinoa: A nutrient-dense grain that is high in protein and fiber.

Uses: Salads, side dishes, soups, and as a base for grain bowls.

Corn: Used in various forms, including cornmeal, corn flour, and polenta.

Uses: Cornbread, tortillas, grits, and as a thickener.

Oats: Naturally gluten-free, but check for cross-contamination.

Uses: Breakfast oatmeal, granola, baking.

Buckwheat: Despite its name, buckwheat is gluten-free and nutritious.

Uses: Pancakes, soba noodles, porridge.

Amaranth: A small, protein-rich grain.

Uses: Porridge, baking, and as a side dish.

Millet: A mild-flavored grain that cooks quickly.

Uses: Breakfast cereals, pilafs, baking.

Teff: A tiny grain that is a staple in Ethiopian cuisine.

Uses: Injera (Ethiopian flatbread), porridge, baking.

Sorghum: A hearty grain that can be used in various dishes.

Uses: Porridge, baking, and as a whole grain side dish.

Gluten-Free Flours: Various flours can be used in baking and cooking, including almond flour, coconut flour, chickpea flour, tapioca flour, and potato flour.

Recipes and Meal Plans for a Wheat-Free Diet

Breakfast Options

1. **Quinoa Porridge**: Cook quinoa with almond milk, sweeten with honey, and top with fresh berries and nuts.
2. **Oatmeal**: Use certified gluten-free oats and cook with your favorite milk. Add fruits, nuts, and seeds for extra nutrition.
3. **Smoothie Bowls**: Blend your favorite fruits with spinach, almond milk, and a scoop of protein powder. Top with granola made from gluten-free oats and seeds.

Lunch Ideas

1. **Rice Salad**: Combine cooked brown rice with chopped vegetables, beans, and a light vinaigrette.
2. **Lettuce Wraps**: Use large lettuce leaves to wrap grilled chicken, avocado, and veggies.

3. **Corn Tortilla Tacos**: Fill gluten-free corn tortillas with black beans, salsa, avocado, and shredded lettuce.

Dinner Recipes

1. **Stuffed Bell Peppers**: Fill bell peppers with a mixture of quinoa, black beans, tomatoes, and spices. Bake until tender.
2. **Gluten-Free Pasta**: Use rice or corn-based pasta and top with marinara sauce and vegetables.
3. **Grilled Salmon with Millet**: Serve grilled salmon over a bed of cooked millet with a side of steamed broccoli.

Snacks and Desserts

1. **Energy Balls**: Mix gluten-free oats, almond butter, honey, and chocolate chips. Roll into balls and refrigerate.
2. **Fruit and Nut Bars**: Combine dried fruits, nuts, and seeds with a bit of honey and press into a baking dish. Chill and cut into bars.

3. **Coconut Flour Cookies**: Use coconut flour to bake cookies with almond butter, honey, and dark chocolate chips.

Sample Meal Plan

Day 1

- **Breakfast**: Quinoa porridge with berries and nuts.
- **Lunch**: Lettuce wraps with grilled chicken and avocado.
- **Dinner**: Stuffed bell peppers with quinoa and black beans.
- **Snack**: Energy balls.

Day 2

- **Breakfast**: Smoothie bowl with gluten-free granola.
- **Lunch**: Rice salad with vegetables and beans.
- **Dinner**: Grilled salmon with millet and steamed broccoli.
- **Snack**: Fruit and nut bars.

Day 3

- **Breakfast**: Oatmeal with fruits and nuts.
- **Lunch**: Corn tortilla tacos with black beans and salsa.
- **Dinner**: Gluten-free pasta with marinara sauce and vegetables.
- **Snack**: Coconut flour cookies.

Challenges and Solutions

Adopting a wheat-free lifestyle can present various social and practical challenges. Here are some common challenges and strategies to overcome them.

Addressing Social and Practical Challenges of a Wheat-Free Lifestyle

Social Situations: Attending parties, family gatherings, and social events can be challenging when avoiding wheat.

Solution: Inform the host about your dietary needs in advance. Offer to bring a gluten-free dish to share.

Dining Out: Finding wheat-free options at restaurants can be difficult.

Solution: Research restaurants with gluten-free menus. Ask the server about wheat-free options and potential cross-contamination.

Traveling: Maintaining a wheat-free diet while traveling requires planning.

Solution: Pack gluten-free snacks for the journey. Research gluten-free restaurants and grocery stores at your destination.

Cross-Contamination: Avoiding cross-contamination at home and in shared kitchens is crucial.

Solution: Use separate utensils, cutting boards, and toasters for gluten-free foods. Clean surfaces thoroughly to avoid contamination.

Tips for Dining Out and Traveling While Avoiding Wheat

Dining Out

1. **Choose the Right Restaurant**: Opt for restaurants that offer gluten-free menus or are known for accommodating dietary restrictions.
2. **Ask Questions**: Don't hesitate to ask the server about ingredients and preparation methods. Ensure there is no cross-contamination.
3. **Simplify Your Order**: Choose simple dishes like grilled meats, salads, and steamed vegetables that are less likely to contain hidden wheat.
4. **Bring Your Own**: If you're unsure about the menu, consider bringing a small snack or meal that you know is safe.

Traveling

1. **Plan Ahead**: Research gluten-free options at your destination. Look for

hotels with kitchen facilities so you can prepare your meals.

2. **Pack Smart**: Bring a variety of gluten-free snacks, such as nuts, seeds, dried fruits, and gluten-free bars.
3. **Communicate Your Needs**: Inform airlines, hotels, and tour operators about your dietary requirements in advance.
4. **Use Technology**: Apps like "Find Me Gluten Free" can help you locate gluten-free restaurants and stores.

Living a wheat-free life requires knowledge, planning, and adaptability. By identifying hidden sources of wheat, using suitable substitutes, and addressing social and practical challenges, you can maintain a wheat-free diet and improve your health. With the right strategies, navigating a wheat-free lifestyle can be manageable and rewarding, leading to better well-being and quality of life.

Chapter 8

The Path to Recovery and Optimal Health

Detoxing from Wheat

Detoxing from wheat involves eliminating it from your diet and allowing your body to adjust. This process can lead to improved health and well-being. Here's how to do it effectively.

Steps for Eliminating Wheat from the Diet and Detoxifying the Body

1. **Educate Yourself**: Understand the sources of wheat and gluten in your diet. Learn to read food labels and identify hidden sources of wheat.
2. **Plan Your Meals**: Create a meal plan that includes wheat-free foods. Focus on whole, minimally processed foods such as fruits, vegetables, lean proteins, and gluten-free grains.

3. **Remove Temptations**: Clear your pantry and kitchen of wheat-containing products. Replace them with gluten-free alternatives.
4. **Gradual Elimination**: If going cold turkey is too challenging, gradually reduce your wheat intake. Start by cutting out obvious sources like bread and pasta, then eliminate hidden sources.
5. **Stay Hydrated**: Drink plenty of water to help flush out toxins from your body. Proper hydration supports overall health and aids in the detoxification process.
6. **Increase Fiber Intake**: Consuming fiber-rich foods like vegetables, fruits, and gluten-free grains helps support digestive health and promotes the elimination of waste.
7. **Support Your Gut**: Include probiotic-rich foods like yogurt, kefir, and fermented vegetables to support gut health during the transition.

8. **Monitor Your Progress**: Keep track of your symptoms, energy levels, and overall well-being as you eliminate wheat from your diet.

Managing Withdrawal Symptoms and Cravings

1. **Understand Withdrawal Symptoms**: When you stop eating wheat, you might experience withdrawal symptoms such as headaches, fatigue, irritability, and cravings. These symptoms usually last for a few days to a few weeks as your body adjusts.
2. **Stay Busy**: Engage in activities that distract you from cravings, such as exercise, hobbies, or spending time with friends and family.
3. **Healthy Snacks**: Keep healthy, gluten-free snacks on hand to curb cravings. Nuts, seeds, fruits, and vegetables are great options.
4. **Stay Positive**: Remind yourself of the benefits of quitting wheat and focus

on your health goals. Positive thinking can help you stay motivated.

5. **Get Support**: Join a support group or find a friend or family member who can help you stay on track and offer encouragement.

6. **Mindful Eating**: Practice mindful eating by paying attention to your hunger and fullness cues. This can help you avoid overeating and manage cravings.

7. **Gradual Reduction**: If cravings are intense, gradually reduce your wheat intake rather than stopping abruptly. This can make the transition smoother.

Long-Term Health Benefits

Quitting wheat can lead to significant health improvements. Here are some case studies and scientific evidence supporting the benefits of a wheat-free diet.

Case Studies of Individuals Who Experienced Health Transformations After Quitting Wheat

Case Study 1: Murphy's Weight Loss Journey

Murphy, a 45-year-old man, struggled with obesity and related health issues. After deciding to quit wheat, he noticed a gradual weight loss and increased energy levels. Within six months, Murphy lost 30 pounds, his blood sugar levels stabilized, and he felt more energetic. Murphy's journey shows how eliminating wheat can support weight loss and improve metabolic health.

Case Study 2: Louise's Digestive Health

Louise, a 38-year-old teacher, suffered from chronic bloating, gas, and irregular bowel movements. After eliminating wheat from her diet, Louise's digestive symptoms significantly improved. She no longer experienced daily discomfort and felt more comfortable and less bloated. Louise's case highlights the digestive benefits of a wheat-free diet.

Case Study 3: Peter's Mental Clarity

Peter, a 29-year-old software developer, struggled with brain fog and difficulty concentrating. After removing wheat from his diet, Peter noticed a marked improvement in his mental clarity and focus. He felt more alert and productive at work. Peter's experience demonstrates the cognitive benefits of eliminating wheat.

Scientific Evidence Supporting the Benefits of a Wheat-Free Diet

1. **Weight Management**: Studies have shown that individuals who eliminate wheat and gluten from their diets often experience weight loss and improved body composition. A gluten-free diet can reduce inflammation, improve insulin sensitivity, and promote healthier eating habits.

2. **Digestive Health**: Research indicates that a gluten-free diet can benefit individuals with celiac disease, non-celiac gluten sensitivity, and irritable bowel syndrome (IBS). Removing wheat can reduce digestive symptoms, improve nutrient absorption, and enhance gut health.

3. **Mental Health**: Some studies suggest that a gluten-free diet can improve mental health outcomes, particularly in individuals with gluten sensitivity. Reduced inflammation and improved gut health can positively impact mood, cognitive function, and overall mental well-being.

4. **Autoimmune Conditions**: A gluten-free diet is essential for managing celiac disease, an autoimmune condition triggered by gluten. Additionally, some research suggests that eliminating gluten may benefit other autoimmune disorders by reducing inflammation and immune system activation.

Maintaining a Balanced Diet

Ensuring nutritional adequacy while avoiding wheat is crucial for long-term health. Here's how to maintain a balanced, wheat-free diet.

Ensuring Nutritional Adequacy While Avoiding Wheat

1. **Diversify Your Diet**: Include a wide variety of foods to ensure you get all the necessary nutrients. Focus on fruits, vegetables, lean proteins, gluten-free grains, nuts, seeds, and healthy fats.
2. **Monitor Nutrient Intake**: Pay attention to essential nutrients that might be lacking in a wheat-free diet, such as fiber, B vitamins, iron, and magnesium. Incorporate foods rich in these nutrients to meet your dietary needs.
3. **Use Fortified Foods**: Choose gluten-free products that are fortified with essential nutrients like iron,

folate, and fiber to help fill any nutritional gaps.

4. **Consider Supplements**: If needed, consider taking supplements to ensure you get adequate amounts of key nutrients. Consult with a healthcare provider or a registered dietitian before starting any supplements.

Incorporating Diverse, Whole Foods for Optimal Health

Fruits and Vegetables: Aim to fill half your plate with fruits and vegetables. They are rich in vitamins, minerals, fiber, and antioxidants.

Examples: Berries, leafy greens, citrus fruits, bell peppers, carrots, and broccoli.

Lean Proteins: Include a variety of protein sources to support muscle health and overall well-being.

Examples: Chicken, turkey, fish, tofu, legumes, and eggs.

Healthy Fats: Incorporate sources of healthy fats to support brain health, hormone production, and nutrient absorption.

Examples: Avocado, nuts, seeds, olive oil, and fatty fish.

Gluten-Free Grains: Choose gluten-free grains that provide essential nutrients and fiber.

Examples: Quinoa, brown rice, millet, amaranth, and gluten-free oats.

Nuts and Seeds: Include a variety of nuts and seeds in your diet for additional fiber, protein, and healthy fats.

Examples: Almonds, chia seeds, flaxseeds, sunflower seeds, and walnuts.

Dairy or Dairy Alternatives: Ensure you get enough calcium and vitamin D from dairy or fortified non-dairy alternatives.

Examples: Greek yogurt, almond milk, and soy milk.

Sample Balanced Meal Plan

Day 1

- **Breakfast**: Greek yogurt with gluten-free granola, fresh berries, and a drizzle of honey.
- **Lunch**: Quinoa salad with mixed greens, cherry tomatoes, cucumber, avocado, and grilled chicken, dressed with olive oil and lemon juice.
- **Dinner**: Baked salmon with a side of roasted sweet potatoes and steamed broccoli.
- **Snack**: Apple slices with almond butter.

Day 2

- **Breakfast**: Smoothie made with spinach, banana, almond milk, and a scoop of protein powder.
- **Lunch**: Lentil soup with a side of gluten-free bread.

- **Dinner**: Stir-fried tofu with mixed vegetables (bell peppers, carrots, snow peas) served over brown rice.
- **Snack**: Carrot sticks with hummus.

Day 3

- **Breakfast**: Oatmeal made with gluten-free oats, topped with sliced almonds, raisins, and a sprinkle of cinnamon.
- **Lunch**: Turkey and avocado lettuce wraps with a side of quinoa salad.
- **Dinner**: Grilled shrimp with a side of millet and a mixed vegetable medley.
- **Snack**: Handful of mixed nuts.

Detoxing from wheat and maintaining a balanced diet can lead to significant health improvements. By eliminating wheat, managing withdrawal symptoms, and focusing on diverse, whole foods, you can achieve optimal health and well-being. The journey to a wheat-free life requires commitment and knowledge, but the benefits are well worth the effort. Embrace the changes, stay informed, and enjoy the path to better health.

Conclusion

Call to Action

Summarizing the Book's Key Messages

Throughout this book, we've explored the profound impact that wheat has on our health. From its historical significance to its modern-day role in the obesity epidemic and chronic diseases, wheat has undergone significant transformations. Here are the key messages from each chapter:

The History of Wheat: From Ancient Grain to Modern Menace

Wheat has evolved from a nutritious ancient grain to a heavily processed staple in the modern diet.

The Green Revolution introduced high-yield dwarf wheat, which significantly altered wheat's nutritional profile.

Understanding Wheat Addiction

Wheat can be addictive, stimulating appetite and cravings through biochemical pathways.

Recognizing the signs of wheat addiction is crucial for making informed dietary choices.

The Hidden Dangers of Modern Wheat

   a. Modern wheat has lost much of its nutritional value compared to ancient varieties.
   b. Refined wheat products contribute to chronic diseases such as obesity, diabetes, and heart disease.
   c. The gluten controversy highlights the various health issues associated with wheat consumption.

2. **Wheat's Role in the Obesity Epidemic**
   a. Wheat's high caloric density and glycemic index contribute

to weight gain and insulin resistance.

b. Reducing wheat consumption can help break the cycle of obesity and promote weight loss.

3. **Wheat and Mental Health**

a. Wheat consumption can negatively affect cognitive function, mental clarity, and mood.

b. Eliminating wheat can improve mental health and alleviate symptoms of depression and anxiety.

4. **The Inflammation Connection**

a. Wheat triggers inflammatory processes in the body, contributing to chronic inflammation and related diseases.

b. An anti-inflammatory, wheat-free diet can reduce inflammation and improve overall health.

5. **Navigating a Wheat-Free Life**
    a. Identifying hidden sources of wheat and finding suitable substitutes are essential for maintaining a wheat-free diet.
    b. Practical tips for dining out and traveling can help you stay wheat-free in various situations.
6. **The Path to Recovery and Optimal Health**
    a. Detoxing from wheat and managing withdrawal symptoms can lead to significant health improvements.
    b. A balanced, wheat-free diet supports long-term health and well-being.

Encouraging Readers to Take Control of Their Health by Reducing or Eliminating Wheat from Their Diet

Taking control of your health by reducing or eliminating wheat from your diet can lead to profound improvements in your physical and mental well-being. Here are some steps to get started:

1. **Educate Yourself**: Understand the sources of wheat in your diet and learn to identify hidden wheat in processed foods.
2. **Plan and Prepare**: Create meal plans that focus on whole, minimally processed foods. Prepare your meals to ensure they are wheat-free.
3. **Gradual Transition**: If eliminating wheat entirely seems daunting, start by gradually reducing your intake and replacing wheat-based foods with healthier alternatives.
4. **Seek Support**: Join support groups or find friends and family members who

can support your journey. Share your experiences and learn from others.

5. **Monitor Your Progress**: Keep track of your symptoms, energy levels, and overall health as you reduce or eliminate wheat. Celebrate your successes and stay motivated by the positive changes you observe.

6. **Stay Informed**: Continue to educate yourself about nutrition and health. Stay updated on the latest research and recommendations for a wheat-free diet.

By making these changes, you can take control of your health and enjoy the benefits of a wheat-free lifestyle. Improved digestion, better mental clarity, reduced inflammation, and overall well-being are just some of the positive outcomes you can achieve.

Acknowledgements

Writing this book has been a journey of discovery and enlightenment. I am grateful to the many individuals who contributed their knowledge, support, and encouragement along the way.

First and foremost, I would like to thank my family for their unrelenting support and understanding as I dedicated countless hours to research and writing. Your patience and encouragement have been invaluable to me.

I am also deeply grateful to my colleagues in the field of nutrition and health sciences. Your insights and expertise have enriched the content of this book and provided a solid foundation for the information presented.

Special thanks to the individuals who shared their personal stories of health transformation after eliminating wheat from their diets. Your experiences have inspired and motivated many to make positive changes in their lives.

Lastly, I extend my appreciation to the editors, researchers, and publishers who helped bring this book to life. Your dedication and hard work have ensured that this book is a valuable resource for readers seeking to improve their health and well-being.

About the Author

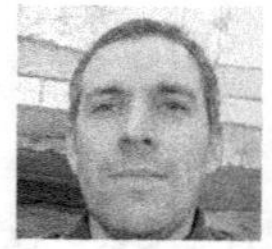 Dr. Myles Watson Collins is a renowned nutritionist and health advocate with over 20 years of experience in the field. He holds a Ph.D. in Nutrition Science and has dedicated his career to researching the impacts of diet on health. Dr. Collins is passionate about educating the public on the benefits of a balanced, whole-foods diet and empowering individuals to take control of their health.

His work has been published in numerous scientific journals, and she is a sought-after speaker at health conferences and seminars. Dr. Collins's approach to nutrition is holistic, focusing on the interplay between diet, lifestyle, and overall well-being.

In addition to his professional achievements, Dr. Collins is an avid cook and enjoys creating nutritious, delicious meals for his family. He believes that healthy eating should be enjoyable and accessible to everyone.

Taking control of your health by reducing or eliminating wheat from your diet is a powerful step towards achieving optimal health. With the knowledge and strategies presented in this book, you are equipped to make informed decisions and embark on a journey of improved well-being. Remember, the path to better health is a continuous process of learning, adapting, and growing. Embrace the changes, stay committed, and enjoy the positive transformation in your life.